Glaucoma Explained

Glaucoma Facts, Diagnosis, Symptoms, Treatment,
Causes, Effects, Alternative Medicines, Therapeutic
Methods, History, Home Remedies, and More!

By Frederick Earlstein

Copyrights and Trademarks

Disclaimer and Legal Notice

Foreword

There is an estimated 3 million Americans who have glaucoma and half of these numbers are not even aware that they are afflicted with the eye disease which robs one of their ability to see. Glaucoma accounts for 9-12% of all instances of partial or sudden blindness.

Glaucoma is the second (to cataracts) leading reason for partial or sudden and total blindness worldwide. Amongst the leading cause of blindness all over the world is atributed to the development of one sort of glaucoma in a patient as reported by the World Health Organization.

The lack of uniformity in defining glaucoma in its various forms is a growing concern for many medical specialists since this eye disease is responsible for an approximate 5.2 million people who have gone blind. Currently, the disease is responsible for blindness in 15% of the world population. Glaucoma is the second leading reason for partial or sudden and total blindness amongst African Americans. Glaucoma is 6 to 8 times more prevalent in African Americans than in Caucasians.

Table of Contents

Introduction

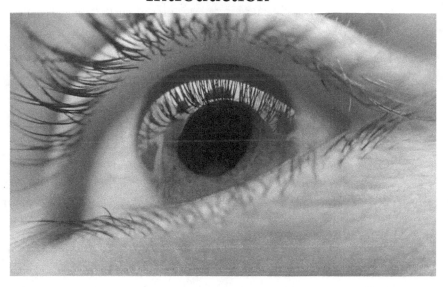

There are presently about 3 million Americans who suffer from glaucoma in one form or another. It is believed that half of these people who are affected by it are not even aware of their plight because there are very little visible or felt indications of glaucoma in a person. Glaucoma is one amongst the leading causes of irreversible blindness in the whole world. There are different types of glaucoma and a number of ways it can affect people.

This degenerative eye disease has affected about 6 million people all over the world. It has also left many individuals sightless in one or both eyes.

This degenerative disease of the eyes first renders partial blindness, which can lead up to total blindness if not detected and treated. The occurrence of glaucoma in a patient gives away very little in terms of symptoms. It could be difficult to identify the onset of glaucoma if you are not aware of how it is manifested.

It is a disease of the eyes which slowly robs an individual of their vision. It does not show apparent during the early stages of the disease so if not caught early the damage to the optic nerve and the loss of vision from glaucoma is irremediable.

Our aim is to reveal more of this occurring disease of the optic nerve and empower the reader to determine what to look out for and what sort of treatments are available. Understanding what the disease a person experiences is the first step to taking back some confidence and control in the situation.

Knowing how you can battle and combat the effect, working around some things, and being able to take charge of some aspects of the disease makes it easier for the patient to deal with any changes and regain some control. There are many ways for us to avoid any damage of contribute to any more by merely finding out more about what to do and what not to do.

Introduction

An ounce of prevention is better than a pound of cure is a saying well suited for anyone who has concerns about their ability to see. With the advent of gadgets and devices that are able to look into the eyes allows us to be at an advantage of being proactive about taking care of our optical health.

Get to know more about the second leading cause of blindness of people, young and old, women and men, and discover what to expect at the doctor's office. Find out about possible telltale signs which may accompany some sorts of glaucoma, be aware of how you can improve your life by making adjustments to your lifestyle, and get to learn about the importance of diet and nutrients needed to maintain optimum eye health and overall wellness.

Chapter One: The Robber of Sight

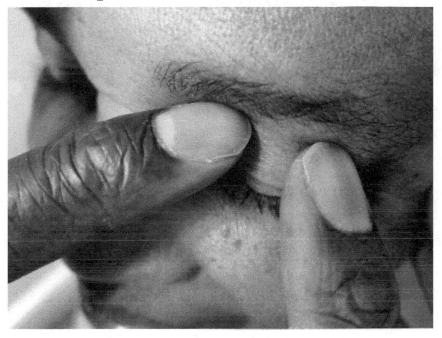

The optic nerve is one of the important components of mechanisms that allow the transition of signals between the eye and the brain. It is the major nerve in our eyes which receive light generated nerve impulses which originate from the retina. The optic nerve does the job of transmitting signals to the brain allowing us to recognize through visualization. These electrical indications received are what we recognize as vision. Glaucoma is a disease that affects the optic nerve limiting the transition of messages between the eyes and the brain. It is the accumulation of fluid behind the eyes that leads to partial or total loss of vision.

Glaucoma is a pretty tricky eye disease to detect and identify because it could, but not always, be associated with intraocular pressure. This is a condition where fluid buildup in the eye is at an increased pressure within it. It is usually this elevated pressure which causes damage to the optic nerve.

When a pattern of progressive damage to the optic nerve is accompanied by a slight loss of peripheral vision, glaucoma could be the suspected culprit. Glaucoma, if not detected and given treatment, will likely lead to central vision loss as well as blindness.

There are some cases when glaucoma can develop even with normal eye pressure - this is when the disease is believed to be stemming from poor blood flow and regulation to the optic nerve. Learn more about it as you read the next sections.

Your Eye Exposed - A Worded Diagram

Our eyes are protected and fortified with a thin, white covering called the sclera. This is the supporting wall of the eyes, or the whites of the eye, which leads up to the cornea. Covering the sclera is a fine, clear membrane called the conjunctiva, which stretches out to the edge of the cornea.

The transparent covering over the eyes, which allows light in and functions as the eye's outermost lenses is the cornea. The cornea acts much like a window, as it controls and focuses the light which enters the eye.

The part of the eye which is colored is called the iris. The iris not only defines the color of a person's eyes, it is also responsible for controlling the diameter of the pupil. The iris expands and contracts to allow just the right amount of light into the eye.

Along the inside back of our eye is the sheer lining of tissue is called the retina. The retina is located in close proximity to the optic nerve. Inside the retina are nerve fibers, doing the job of transmitting images to the brain via the optic nerve.

The retina does the job of taking in light. Light which the lens focuses on converts the received light into electric or neural signals. These signals are then transmitted to our brains thereby allowing for visual identification.

The Inner Mechanisms of Your Eye

The aqueous humor or the intraocular fluid is made by the ciliary body and is the clear fluid that fills the front part of our eyes. The aqueous humor streams out by way of the pupil of the eyes. This fluid is taken into a person's bloodstream and through a network of drainage canals, the eye's system of drainage, known as the trabecular meshwork.

The trabecular meshwork is the space between the cornea, the clear part of the eye and the iris, the colored part of the eye. This drainage system of the eye is located at an angle, very near the edge of the iris.

When the drainage is correct, the eye pressure is kept at a normal level. In order for the process to remain constant, the production and streaming of the aqueous humor should be active in order for a person to enjoy optimum visual health.

The intraocular pressure or the inner pressure of the eye relies on the equilibrium of production as well as drainage of the fluid in the eye. The inner pressure can be different throughout the day however; this should remain in a range that is manageable.

The eye drainage system that works properly drains fluids out freely thereby preventing fluid buildup in the eye. A properly operating trabecular meshwork should produce just the right amount of fluid. A healthy eye allows for the proper production and flow of aqueous humor through the eye and drains correctly in the drainage canal.

When Glaucoma Is Present

An eye drainage canal diseased with glaucoma is blocked and the buildup of the aqueous humor is prevented from being drained. This inability to drain the aqueous humor causes buildup in the eye. The buildup of the fluid when prevented from draining properly increases the pressure to the eye. It is the accumulation of the fluid which eventually damages the optic nerve of the individual.

The eye's trabecular meshwork, which is the network of drainage canals in the eye, cannot drain fluid correctly when it becomes clogged. And this is the culprit of most types of glaucoma – when the fluid in the eyes buildup, this causes pressure to increase in the eye and when the pressure gets high, this damages the optic nerve, a sensitive part of the eye which transmits electronic signals to the brain. The failure of transition of electronic signals to the brain results to vision impairment and or blindness.

The body is an amazing machine. Take the eye for example. There are millions of nerve fibers running from the retina all the way to the optic nerve. Millions! These millions of sensitive fibers all converge at the optic disc. When the fluid buildup increases in the eyes, this creates the pressure that causes irreparable damage to the very sensitive nerve fibers. Once these nerve fibers are damaged, the disc of the eyes will start to hollow out, developing a curved or inverted-cup shape. Prolonged increase in the pressure destroys the optic nerve.

Intraocular pressure was once thought to be the main cause of optic nerve damage but it is now clear that there must be other factors involved as well since people with a normal intraocular pressure reading can come up against loss of vision stemming from glaucoma.

Glaucoma typically affects both eyes; however, the pressure of excess fluid usually begins in one eye at the onset. The pressure of the extra fluid causes gradual destruction indicated by changes in visual ability which leads to vision loss. Peripheral vision, or side vision, is what usually gives indication to the deteriorating vision.

The changes in the vision of one suffering from glaucoma is so subtle that it may not even be noticed at first, but will become more apparent with the passing of time. If not diagnosed and treated the partial blindness can lead up to central vision loss; this is when the direct vision of a person is compromised.

Glaucoma by the Numbers

(Status of Glaucoma in U.S. and the world, Stats of Glaucoma by age, Stats of Glaucoma by other factors)

There are about 6 million people the world over who suffer from this very misunderstood disease of the eyes. Unfortunately most people who suffer from it are not even aware of having glaucoma. It is the leading cause of progressive or sudden blindness in people and can affect anyone.

Sadly, an approximate ten percent of glaucoma patients, even after receiving proper care and medication, still undergo loss of vision. There is currently no known cure for glaucoma nor can one regain the vision they have lost once gone. Cataracts are the foremost culprit for causing blindness amongst African Americans. It is also 6 to 8 times more likely to be seen amongst African Americans than in Caucasians. Open angle glaucoma, the most common form of glaucoma is responsible for 19% of all blindness in African Americans in contrast to 6% accounting for blindness in Caucasians.

People who are diabetic, those who are over 60 years old are some of the people who fall under the high risk group of people who could develop one form of glaucoma or another.

Others considered to be in the high risk group are those who have family members who have been diagnosed with glaucoma or other eye diseases which may pave the way for glaucoma.

Alarmingly, those whose chances for developing or having glaucoma are mostly unaware of the group of eye diseases which lead to blindness - and that encompasses all humans 16% African Americans out of over a thousand interviewed said they were not aware or familiar with glaucoma whilst 9% Caucasian interviewees said they were not familiar with the disease.

Sadly, glaucoma is the most prevalent cause of avoidable, irreparable vision loss across the world with primary open angle glaucoma accounting for an average 12% of blindness worldwide. It is said to be the one of the leading causes of blindness amongst the Chinese.

The promise of preventing further loss of vision can be remedied and stopped through surgery and can also be deterred through treatment and medication. Diagnosis is very important to stop the condition from progressing. It is the initial need to be able to prevent complete blindness and preservation of visual ability.

Although older people are likelier and have a higher chance for glaucoma, no one is spared from the risk of developing the degenerative, incurable eye disease. From babies to senior citizens, everyone is potentially at risk for contracting glaucoma.

Even though older individuals possess higher risk of developing glaucoma, there is an approximate 1 baby out of every 10,000 newborns delivered in the United States alone who can be birthed with glaucoma. Whilst glaucoma seems to target young adults in general, there are a greater number of young African Americans who develop glaucoma.

The sort of glaucoma most prevalent is open-angle glaucoma and almost has no symptoms that give indication to the disease. The pressure typically does not cause pain. There is basically no discomfort felt by the individual related to increasing fluid retention behind the eyes.

A patient, on the throes of glaucoma, could compensate for vision loss by turning their heads from side to side so that they can see and focus better on an image. Others could unknowingly suffer and may not even notice the deterioration of vision until a significant part of their vision is lost. Prior to full disclosure upon diagnosis, peripheral vision loss is usually compromised and even then the damage would have already been done.

Anyone can develop and suffer from glaucoma. It spares no one from babies to individuals who are advanced in age. However, there are some individuals who are more prone to developing glaucoma.

People who are over 60 years old run a higher risk than younger people. Those of Asian, Hispanic or African heritage also run a higher risk. People who are related, at least to the second to third degree, to a person who has or had glaucoma is another cluster of people susceptible to it.

Who are those with the higher likelihood of developing glaucoma? Those who have been diagnosed to be either near sighted and people who have been determined to be farsighted are some of those individuals. Individuals, young or old, who have myopic or hyperopic eye conditions, are the ones most prone to glaucoma.

When tests have been conducted on an individual and the reading of increased pressure in the eyes is the conclusion, this could be the onset of glaucoma. When the central cornea has been determined to have thinned can be another indication of glaucoma onset.

When it has been determined that steroid medication has been used or if the presence, an event or after events of an eye injury are all conditions which increase the risk of glaucoma in a patient.

All sorts of glaucoma identified can cause damage to the optic nerve attributing to too much of the blindness experienced in the world today. Only early detection and treatment can stop the progress of the damaging eye disease.

If arrested at an early onset, medicine, therapy and treatment is available to deter from any further destruction to the optic nerve. Not everyone experiencing increased eye pressure (IOP) necessarily get glaucoma. There are some individuals who are able to tolerate higher levels of pressure in the eyes than others do. Not to mention that a normal eye pressure to one may to too high for another.

The level for each one is different. A person who develops glaucoma will depend on the pressure level your optic nerve can withstand without causing damage to it. No two people are the same therefore, it is best to get professional advice rather than comparing your symptoms to someone who has seen one and been diagnosed.

Ask your GP or ophthalmologist about a comprehensive dilated eye exam. It will detail and reveal any present risk factors associated with glaucoma and other eye diseases that may lead to glaucoma. This exam will show if there is thinning of the cornea, high eye pressure as well as any abnormalities in the optic nerve.

Chapter Two: Different Types of Glaucoma

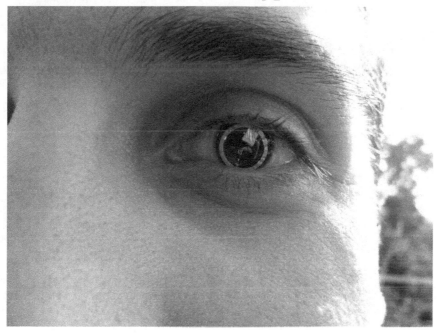

The two cases of common glaucoma, open-angle and angle-closure, are each marked by elevated pressure inside a patient's eye and accounts for at least ninety – percent of all cases of glaucoma. Variants of open-angle and angle-closure glaucoma include Uveitic Glaucoma, Neovascular Glaucoma, Secondary Glaucoma, Pseudoexfoliative Glaucoma, Traumatic Glaucoma, Pigmentary Glaucoma, Irido Corneal Endothelial Syndrome (ICE). You'll get to learn

Types of Glaucoma

Open - Angle Glaucoma

Open-angle glaucoma is caused by the gradual clogging of the eye's drainage canals. This can increased IOP. Most people who have open-angle glaucoma do not notice any changes in their vision initially and feel fine.

The intraocular pressure or IOP rises when fluid can't drain out of the eye. The problem of clogging happens further inside the eyes drainage canals. This condition develops gradually and is considered a condition for life that will need maintenance and regular monitoring. Open-angle glaucoma typically responds well to treatment and medication as long as it is arrested immediately.

The upside to this condition is that if a person gets their eyes checked regularly, detecting the condition early and receiving the proper treatment can preserve the vision of the patient. Otherwise, it can lead to total blindness.

Angle-closure Glaucoma

Angle-closure glaucoma is a less common form of glaucoma that is caused by the blocking of eye drainage canals and can rapidly develop. There are some symptoms usually because of noticeable damage to vision or the eyes. It is imperative to get immediate medical attention with angle-closure glaucoma.

Symptoms of angle-closure glaucoma may include the appearance of rainbow-colored circles around bright lights, hazy or blurred vision, severe eye pain and head aches, vomiting or nausea accompanied by severe pain in the eye, and sudden loss of sight.

Congenital Glaucoma

Congenital Glaucoma is a type of glaucoma which occurs in babies when there is incorrect or incomplete development of the baby's eye drainage canals during the prenatal stage. If uncomplicated, microsurgery can correct the structural defects of the trabecular meshwork while other cases can be treated with medication.

When a patient suffers from Normal-Tension Glaucoma the optic nerve is damaged even though the eye pressure is not as high. Experts are still in the dark as to why some people's optic nerves get damaged even though they have almost near normal pressure levels. It is a unique condition in which optic nerve damage and vision loss have occurred regardless of normal pressure inside the eye.

The incident of normal-tension glaucoma have different statistics around the world, however it seems that it has a high percentage among Japanese patients. In the United States, up to 15-25% of patients with open-angle glaucoma go through normal-tension glaucoma. Routine eye examinations with an ophthalmologist are going to be very important since patients with normal-tension glaucoma do not experience any early symptoms of the condition.

Being at Risk

A person is at an increased risk for glaucoma if there is history of it in the family. Being of a certain heritage is also a factor; African Americans, Latinos or Asians are seen to be more prone to the eye disease especially people who have been diagnosed diabetic. There is also a high likelihood of open-angle glaucoma if a patient has cardiovascular disease. The risk of glaucoma also heightens with the advancement in age.

What to Expect at the Ophthalmologist

Glaucoma and optic nerve abnormalities are inherited, and your ophthalmologist will want to know if there is a history of these in your family. You will be asked of any recent trauma to the eyes or exposure to toxic chemicals which may impede your visual acuity.

Your ophthalmologist will inquire about any recent illnesses, current use of medications and which kinds, including use of steroids. You will also be asked about history of your vision, any migraine episodes, nearsightedness or myopia.

You will also be asked about any conditions of the blood (high blood, low blood pressures, recent blood loss, and/r bleeding disorders). Sleep apnea, thyroid disease and Alzheimer disease would have to be discussed with your GP since all of these have the potential to be associated with normal-tension glaucoma.

Expect to sit for the eye the examination. The front of your eyes, including your cornea, anterior chamber, iris, and lens, will be examined using the special microscope or the slit lamp. A special contact lens, called a goniolens, is positioned on the patient's eye in order for the ophthalmologist to get a good view of the trabecular meshwork.

A complete treatment is basically made up of 100 spots positioned over the whole trabecular meshwork. This treatment may be divided between 2 sessions. Each session will consist of 50 spots over each half of the trabecular meshwork. The whole procedure typically lasts 30 minutes or less and is relatively painless.

If trabeculoplasty is successful, IOP is usually lessened but this decrease in IOP is not usually permanent, unfortunately. This decrease in IOP may last up to 3-5 years following a trabeculoplasty procedure, if the procedure is successful. After the trabeculoplasty, the eye doctor will prescribe medicine to avoid inflammation while the patient continue's taking glaucoma medicine.

Trabeculectomy may be recommended in severe patient cases with progressive vision loss. During a trabeculectomy exam, the ophthalmologist makes an alternate drainage channel in the patient's eye to increase the flow of aqueous humor fluid from the eye. This helps in lowering the IOP.

Follow-up for Normal-Tension Glaucoma

If a person has normal-tension glaucoma, they will have to have regular follow-up visits with their ophthalmologist in order to monitor any progression of the condition. Follow-up visits are usually scheduled every 3-6 months.

Normal-tension glaucoma cannot be averted but with regular eye exams given by an ophthalmologist, any further progression of the degenerative condition can be avoided.

Other Types of Glaucoma

Secondary Gloucoma isn't like POAG glaucoma when the underlying cause of elevated IOP is made right and helps return proper pressure levels. Once an optic damage has taken place there is no repairing or reversing the condition. But this should even out when normal pressure is achieved.

Secondary glaucoma can develop as a result of other pre-existing medical conditions in a patient. For example, a severe sort of glaucoma called neovascular glaucoma can be a result of poorly controlled diabetes. This disease accounts for 1/3 of the cases of NVG which is much higher in diabetic patients who have diabetic retinopathy. The numbers of NVG in diabetic patients go up even more if they have an eye procedure. Undergoing lensectomy or vitrectomy increases the odds of developing NVG.

Other types of glaucoma can sometimes be accompanied with cataract, certain eye tumors, or when the eye is inflamed or irritated by a condition called uveitis. Uveitis is an inflammation of the middle layer of the eye consisting of the iris, choroid and ciliary body. Exposure to toxic chemical like pesticides, and industrial acid can result to uveitis. Many cases of uveitis are chronic and glaucoma is one possible complication of the condition and if not arrested immediately this can lead to permanent loss of vision.

Uveitis can be caused by a number of things including bacterial, viral and fungal infections. However there are many cases of uveitis with unknown or undetectable origins.

Smoking is said to be one risk factor for uveitis as cigarette smoke contains components that aggregate inflammation inside blood vessels and contribute to the disruption of the immune system. Doctors would usually prescribe pupil dilating drops to lessen pain and discomfort to eyes in addition to steroids. The patient may also be prescribed with eyes drops which would help lower the IOP if high eye pressure is detected stemming from uveitis.

On occasion, secondary ocular hypertension can result from poor positioning of an artificial lens inserted into the eye of a cataract patient. Sometimes it is required that a lens be inserted in the anterior chamber instead of the posterior chamber and this happens support is not sufficient in the existing lens capsule after a delicate and complicated cataract surgery.

It is probable for these lenses to block the passage of aqueous fluid through the pupil which may result in a secondary angle closure. An iridectomy from a peripheral angle is then made at the time of the lens being inserted. In addition patients who have had cataracts removed but had no lens inserted can also be a cause for secondary glaucoma.

Neovascular glaucoma is still a therapeutic challenge which baffles. The key elements to preventing a visually horrible outcome of this blinding eye disease is early detection and prophylactic treatment focused on the retina.

There are times when glaucoma is developed by a person after undergoing other unrelated eye surgeries or surgeries performed because of serious sudden eye injuries. Steroid drugs given to a patient to treat an eye irritation can trigger glaucoma in some people.

One sort of secondary glaucoma is Pseudoexfoliation Glaucoma. This is what happens when there is extra material produced then eventually shed off inside of the internal eye structures which results to the blockage of the meshwork giving the same result of slowing down the aqueous fluid drainage process.

Another form of secondary glaucoma is Pigmentary Glaucoma. This happens when the pigment giving color to the iris begins to shed off, when this damage starts the flakes that are shed blocks and obstructs the meshwork which in turn slows down fluid drainage. This makes buildup of the aqueous fluid to increase the pressure in the eyes.

Depending on the cause of these secondary glaucomas, treatment of these conditions would include medicines. There is also a possible discussion on laser surgery, or conventional or other surgeries aimed to arrest the progression of glaucoma.

Chapter Three: Signs and Symptoms, Diagnosis and Treatments

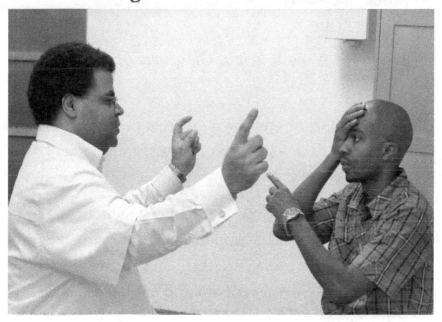

Glaucoma typically does not have any symptoms at the onset of fluid buildup. It takes a while for any physical manifestation to become felt, or noticed by an individual who has been suffering from it. The problem with glaucoma is that it is usually too late for the patient to get proper treatment or at least maintenance once impairment is apparent. We need to know that vision damage due to glaucoma is irreversible.

There is no cure to glaucoma. However, if caught early there are ways to stave off any more damage, which we will be discussing further later in the book.

How Do I know If I Have Glaucoma – Symptoms?

The grave problem about glaucoma is that once the damage starts it will just get worse, without proper treatment.

Glaucoma slowly robs one of their ability to see, and with no usual tell-tale signs to indicate the disease being present. Without diagnosis there can be no treatment, and treatment is the only thing that can help stop this disease from causing further damage.

Regular eye examinations are the only silver lining to this bleak and degenerative serious eye condition. Only when a person, especially those who are more prone to glaucoma than others, gets routine eye examinations are they able to fight off the onset of glaucoma proactively.

A person could go through life and suffer from this blinding disease without given clue to it ravaging their

eyesight. They are only clued in when they experience vision
impairment or total loss of vision.

It is why it is very important for individuals to get
screened on a regular basis. Those predisposed to the
disease are encouraged to get tested even more frequently
with a strong recommendation extended to those who have
a family history of glaucoma.

Benefits of Screening for Glaucoma

A disease model was created to be able to make an
intelligent assumption of the extensiveness of the disease as
it prevails in different countries of the world. Although the
model is still weak given the difficulty in finding any
outwardly symptoms of glaucoma, the purpose of getting
this simple disease model created is to be able to keep track
of the impact of glaucoma on a global scale. This WHO
project for the prevention of blindness not only aims to keep
numbers in countries but it's purpose is also to provide a
more updated and more correct record of information
related to the condition from a population-based assessment
in some countries.

Glaucoma has been categorized to come in different times of a person's life, with relation to ethnicity, age and gender. In each of the nine regions where studies were developed, it was determined that primary open-angle glaucoma, or POAG, is four times higher in amongst people of African ancestry than it is in Caucasians.

Studies also indicated that there is a higher prevalence of glaucoma in women than in men. The prevalence of primary angle-closure glaucoma is also more prevalent in women than in men with a ratio of 1:3 (men: women). Asians have also been seen to develop one form of glaucoma or another more than Caucasians at any age.

Getting examined on a regular basis is vital to all individuals. It is especially more so important for those who are predisposed to the disease to get examined more. There are particular heritages and ancestry who are more prone to the blinding eye disease than others. Those of African descent as well as Asians have been seen to be more prone to glaucoma than those of Caucasian heritage.

The implications of the disease in terms of disability and the growing numbers became a cause of global concern and it was deemed necessary to investigate this seemingly asymptomatically eye disease that has continued to be the culprit of 15% of blindness worldwide.

Because of the alarmingly growing numbers of blindness caused by glaucoma the WHO began to take in global estimates zeroing in on the most commonly seen form of glaucoma in sufferers. The proportion of vision loss perpetrated by glaucoma gave outstanding results with 6.7%-21% in Denmark, Germany, Iceland, Chile, the United States of America and the United Kingdom. 22% of glaucoma sufferers were registered in 17 African and Asian countries, including the countries of Turkey and Peru. The results show that 10-15% of the blindness worldwide is attributed to glaucoma.

How Often Should I Get Screened?

Everyone else should have their eyes checked at least once every five years, whether they think they need to or not, to make sure that all is on the up and up with their eyes. This is all the more important for people showing some signs that may indicate one form of glaucoma or another.

No matter how sneaky glaucoma can be, it is important to remember that for some kinds of glaucoma, clues like hazy vision, rainbow ring colors around lights, peripheral vision loss are advanced indications of one form of eye disease or another.

It is wiser to practice an ounce of prevention than to employ a pound of cure in the long run. There are now available machines, devices and technology that have been developed for the purposes of reducing the incidences of blindness.

The use of potent herbal extracts is used commercially in eye drops and the pool of eye experts, ophthalmologists and technicians abound with skill and ability to detect anomalies in the eyes. Since glaucoma is relatively associated with age, it does not escape the fact that anyone can suffer from glaucoma at any given time of their lives. Here is a table of recommended eye examination intervals as provided by the American Academy of Ophthalmology.

From Age twenty to twenty nine; it is advised that individuals with family members who suffer from glaucoma as well as individuals of African descent be given an eye examination at least once every three to five years.

From thirty to thirty nine age group especially those people who have family with glaucoma as well as those of African descent should make an appointment and undergo an eye examination at least every two to four years, while other individuals, not under any of the categories mentioned, should have an eye exam at least twice within a period of four years.

By age 40 until 64, everybody, regardless of age, gender or ethnicity should be tested once at least in a period of two to four years. Once an individual reaches their 60th milestone, they should go in for an eye examination once in a span of one to two years. People regardless of gender or ethnicity, upon reaching 60 years of age is to be tested at least once a year, at a minimum.

Routine screening is mandatory eye examinations because glaucoma typically develops with no apparent symptoms. Damaged caused by it cannot be regained nor can it be reversed. Therefore, in the advocacy to prevent vision loss and to preserve vision, glaucoma has to be detected, diagnosed and treated early. It is also imperative for individuals to be monitored for glaucoma periodically as advised above.

Those who suffer from glaucoma, no matter what age they are, need to understand that this is a lifelong disease that will need to be monitored and treated. If a glaucoma patient complies with appointed visits to their ophthalmologist, and follow prescribed regimens of medication will offer them the best chance of keeping their vision.

How Physicians Diagnose Glaucoma

Human beings come to accept that we are not infallible and that we all have one thing or another that is not on the up and up. Tests and examinations are available now to determine if a person is unknowingly suffering from glaucoma. Tonometry gives indication of the pressure in the eye of the patient by measuring the firmness of the surface of the eye. The procedure starts off with the eye being administered with localized anesthetic eye drops. One it takes effect the sensor of the tonometer is placed against the front surface of the eye which does the job of emitting a puff off warm air to measure the pressure level of the aqueous fluid in the inner eye.

The eye pressure level of each individual is different. Each has their own unique level of tolerance in terms of pressure level ranges. The normal pressure range is set at 12-22mm Hg but then there are individuals who show pressure readings in this range but still have glaucoma. Glaucoma is usually diagnosed on a patient who shows reading beyond 20 mm Hg.

The Pachymetrytest measures the thickness of the cornea and is a painless exam which begins with anesthetic eye drops. Once the eye is numb the achymeter is lightly rested on the cornea. This is done to see if the thickness of the cornea is affecting the IOP of the patient. Patients with a flimsy cornea could be an indication that the subject may be prone to glaucoma. Determining the thickness of the cornea allows the doctor to interpret the tonometry reading of the patient.

Gonioscopy uses special contact lenses with mirrors placed on the surface of the eye. The mirror of the lens functions such that the doctor is able to look at the eye's interior from different angles and directions. It helps examine the drainage in the eye as well as the angle.

The special lens allows checking if the angle is unobstructed or narrowed. It also gives the doctor a chance to check for other abnormalities like hyperpigmentation or other damage to the angle. Gonioscopy exams can also tell is if there are abnormalities in the blood vessels, the presence of tumor which could be causing blockage. Patients who have narrow angles have a higher likelihood of developing acute angle-closure.

Ophthalmoscopy exams use a head-mounted device, a handheld one or special lenses with a slit lamp to peer into the iris. This is done to see if there is damage to the optic nerve or if there is an indentation or cupping of the disc. Cupping is caused by an increase in IOP. Cupping is also a symptom that a person may have or have developed glaucoma. Ophthalmologists use specialized cameras which can take photographs of the optic nerve, allowing them to compare any changes, if any, happen over time.

Visual field testing provides a map of the visual fields in order to determine any recent or early indications of optic nerve damage due to glaucoma. Random flashes of light are shown at different intensities and the patient is required to push a button when they see a light flash. This is a method of test that creates a computerized mapping of the visual field of the patient. It outlines the portions of the eye which cannot or can see because there are idiosyncratic shifts in the visual field of a patient with glaucoma.

Optical coherence tomography and Confocal laser scanning systems are non-invasive imaging systems which process a 3-D image of the retina and the optic nerve. It indicates the degree of cupping and detects the thicknesses of the retina whilst measuring the ganglion cell layers.

Treatments, Drugs and Medications to Treat Glaucoma

Eye Drop Medication

Even though vision impairment and damage to nerves stemming from glaucoma is not usually reversed. Sufferings from the disease can be overall controlled with the advances of science in relation to studies focused on the effects of glaucoma. Intraocular pressure through treatment and management can normalize the flow of fluid through the vents. This gives a higher likelihood of retarding any more nerve damage, causing eventual blindness
from occurring. There are a number of ways to stave off any more damage from glaucoma from the rare use of prescribed pills to the more often applied use of eye drops and the occasional suggestion of surgery.

There are several types of eye drops available in the pharmaceutical market that is used by patients several times a day to lessen the intraocular pressure in the eye.

Eye drops are the first medication usually used in treating most types of open-angle glaucoma in the United States. Whilst in Europe, it has been observed that eye surgery is usually the first treatment resorted to by glaucoma sufferers in that region. These eye drops help in the increase fluid drainage out of the eyes or it acts like a faucet being shut off and reduces the development of aqueous fluid. For each sort of treatment/therapy, all have their probable complications as well as their benefits.

Blocking or acting against adrenaline-like matter is a beta-adrenergic antagonist working toward treating glaucoma by lessening the development of the aqueous humor. These eye drops were considered to be the gold standard of eye drops against glaucoma. These drops were compared to other eye medication and were considered the best for a time. Some of the medications employed are metipranolol (Optipranolol), carteolol (Ocupress), levobunolol (Betagan) and timolol (Timoptic). These drops are very effective if used once or twice a day.

But it promoted the worsening of other existing conditions and resulted in side effects such as the worsening of emphysema, low blood pressure, bradycardia or slowing down of the heart rate, asthma, impotence and fatigue. It prevented the use of it in some patients.

A beta-adrenergic antagonist called Betaxolol (Betoptic) zeroes in and selectively works on just the eyes, lessening the risks of side effects against the heart and the lings unlike the side effects of other drugs used.

Prostaglandin analogs have the same chemical structure as the body's prostaglandins. These are hormone-like matter which is used in a broad range of workings all throughout the body. The way these Prostaglandin analog eye drops work with glaucoma is by way of the drops increasing the drainage outflow of aqueous fluid from the eye.

Beta-blockers have been replaced by the prostaglandin analogs drops. Prostaglandin analogs are what is typically prescribed for glaucoma which is used just once a day by a glaucoma patient. Some of these medications include tafluprost (Zioptan), bimatoprost (Lumigan), latanoprost (Xalatan), and travoprost (Travatan). The side effect of prostaglandin analogs is pretty minimal in comparison to beta blockers. They are likely to cause redness of the eyes more than other eye drops.

This sort of eye drop medication has lesser side effects to the other parts of the body than beta blockers do. The side effects noticed by users and doctors in prostaglandin analogs are that it changes the color of the iris, as well as darkening and thickening the eyelashes of a user. Additional to these would be emaciated fat around the eyes could be apparent. It could also cause eye inflammation.

Acting like adrenaline is a kind of eye drops called adrenergic agonists. How it works is pretty amazing. It increases the drainage outflow of the eye whilst lessening the development of aqueous fluid by the eye.

Brimonidine (Alphagan) is the most widely prescribed and used adrenergic agonist. But there is at least a 12% of significant allergic reaction localized in the eyes. Other treatment medication of this class of eye drops includes apraclonidine (Iopidine), dipivefrin (Propine), and epinephrine.

Carbonic anhydrase inhibitors are prescribed for glaucoma and it works by lessening the development of aqueous fluid in the eye. These eye drop medications include brinzolamide (Azopt) and dorzolamide (Trusopt) and glaucoma patients are recommended by their physicians to use these drops two or three times a day. On rare occassions carbonic anhydrase inhibitors may also be systematically ingested as pills to eliminate fluids from the body including fluids from the eyes. Oral forms of these medications prescribed for glaucoma patients include acetazolamide (Diamox) and methazolamide (Neptazane).

The use of pill for glaucoma conditions is limited because of its side effects throughout the body. These side effects include numbness or tingling sensations in the lips, arms, and legs, reduction of body potassium, kidney stones, nausea and fatigue.

Parasympathomimetic agents, work in glaucoma by increasing the aqueous outflow from the eye. These eye medication treatments are also known as meiotic due to the fact that they narrow and constrict the pupils, opposing adrenalin-like substances.

Before the advent of prostaglandins and beta-blockers, parasympathomimetics were used for a long time to treat glaucoma. These medications are now rarely used because of the frequency a person needs to use it - three to four times a day - in order to see any effects in the eye.

The side effects of parasympathomimetics include a heightened risk of retinal detachment, blurred vision, small pupil and a painful brow. Pilocarpine, another medication used to treat glaucoma, is currently used to primarily help patients keep their pupil small especially in patients with a specific iris make up, like a plateau iris, or in those with a narrow angle before undergoing laser iridotomy.

An additional class of medications employed to treat acute and sudden forms of glaucoma are osmotic agents. Acute forms of glaucoma come in a form where the eye pressure is at an extreme high even though other treatments have been explored. Some of these medications include mannitol (Osmitrol), administered intravenously through the veins and isosorbide (Ismotic) whichc is orally administered.

Take caution when using these sorts of medication to treat glaucoma because these treatments come with significant side effect that can be immobilizing at its worst.

Side effect of these medications includes congestive heart failure and/or pulmonary edema; these are fluid accumulation in the heart and/or lungs, nausea, kidney problems and bleeding in the brain. These medications are not given to pariens who have liver, heart and kidney problems. These medications are also not given to patients who have uncontrollable diabetes.

When glaucoma patients need more than one sort of medication to control and manage their glaucoma, ophthalmologist would usually write out a prescription of an eye drop that has more than one sort of drug which simplifies the patient's usage of drops.

Some examples of these multiple combination eye drops are the use of both timolol and dorzolamide in the same drop (Cosopt), the use of both timolol and brimonidine in the same drop (Combigan), and the combination of brinzolamide and brimonidine in the same drop (Simbrinza). Both beta-adrenergic antagonists and prostaglandin analogs are combination drops which are available in Europe and Japan butt are not yet approved by the United States Food and Drug Administration (FDA) for use in the US.

There are presently several classes of new glaucoma eye drops in current development. Others are just waiting for a nod from the FDA. These eye drops and medications include rho-kinase inhibitors (Rhopressa), nitrous oxide donating medication combined with prostaglandins (Latanoprostene) and A-1 receptor selective adenosine mimetics (Trabodenoson).

Even though the use of marijuana has been proven to lessen the intraocular pressure, there are available eye drops that serve the same purpose, and do the same job with greater efficacy.

Surgery and Laser Therapy

It is very crucial to keep in mind that there are a lot of patients who are at risk of glaucoma, may already have glaucoma that may have another eye disease like macular degeneration or cataract. Only an ophthalmologist can recognize whether the visual impairment a person experiences is caused by another eye abnormality or if it is glaucoma that is the culprit.

There are patients who get eye exams that show heightened eye pressure and an elevated risk to develop glaucoma, however no precise evidence of damage to eye caused by glaucoma. One condition these patients experience is called ocular hypertension or OHT. This was once termed as glaucoma suspect or pre-glaucoma symptoms.

Patients who have OHT do not complain of loss of field vision but they are more susceptible to the risk of glaucoma. This is because of the elevated intraocular pressure being present in the patient. Elevated pressure and or optic nerve shifts are apparent on imaging and ophthalmoscopy. Many of these patients with OHT need to get treatment. OHT patients will need to be monitored fairly regularly in order to be given the proper treatment they need before the irreversible damages of glaucoma takes hold.

There is a tricky and delicate microsurgery procedure that is employed in the treatment of glaucoma. During the procedure, a tiny portion of the backed up trabecular meshwork is removed to make a passageway and a new pathway of drainage for the aqueous fluid to escape the eye. A tiny bag is collected from conjunctival tissue creating a new drainage system. The fine and clear cover that wraps around the white of the eye is called conjunctival.

The filtering bleb as it is called resembles a raised cystic area which is at the utmost area of the eye beneath the upper lid. This new system of drainage allows for the aqueous fluid to exit the eye and enter the bleb or the bag. The fluid then passes into the capillary circulation of the blood and hence lowers eye pressure in the patient.

The most commonly done surgery on glaucoma patients is the trabeculectomy. If the operation is successful, trabeculectomy is the most effective way to lowering the eye pressure of a glaucoma patient. Glaucoma implants or tubes called aqueous shunt devices are artificial devices that help drainage and lowering the eye pressure.

Essentially these are small plastic tubes which are attached to a reservoir made of plastic. This plate or reservoir is positioned under the conjunctival tissue. The tube extending from the reservoir is then positioned inside the eye making a new route for the aqueous fluid to leave the eye.

The aqueous fluid is collected inside of the reservoir under the conjunctiva making a filtering bleb. This operation can be done as another option to trabeculectomy to patients with specific sorts of glaucoma. There are also mini shunts without a reservoir used to reduce the after surgery chance of pressures being too low as it improves the safety of the procedure.

Minimally-invasive glaucoma surgery, also called MIGS, has been underway in the recent past few years. Different devices like the IStent, the CyPass Micro-Stent, the Trabectome, the Xen glaucoma implant, the Hydrus Microstent, Viscocanaloplasty and the InnFocus Microshunt are either already used in advanced clinical trials or have been approved for the use of humans.

These are alternative surgical methods which are
employed to lower pressure in the eye of a glaucoma patient.
These methods are aimed to create new pathways in the
trabecular meshwork. These operations are much less
invasive than aqueous shunt and trabeculectomy surgeries,
although these may not lower pressure as much.

The surgeon sometimes creates other types of drainage
systems. While glaucoma surgery is frequently effective,
there are complications, like bleeding or infection that could
occur. Surgery is typically the last resort for patients that
display cases of glaucoma which cannot be controlled
otherwise.

There are currently several forms of laser therapy to arrest
and stunt glaucoma. A hole made in the colored part of the
eye or the iris in order for fluid to drain as it should in eyes
with narrow or closed angles is a method of surgery called
Laser Iridotomy. Laser procedures performed only in eyes
with open angles.

Selective laser trabeculoplasty (SLT) and Argon laser
trabeculoplasty are laser surgery procedures done only on
eyes with open angles. These procedures do not in any way
cure glaucoma but are sometimes done in lieu of prescribing
more eye drops of different sorts. This could also be

recommended if a patient has already been using a number
of various eye drops.

There are some situations when this is employed as the
primary or initial therapy for open-angle glaucoma. It is a
procedure that is relatively painless, fast and a safer method
to lower the intraocular pressure. Using anesthetic drops to
numb the eye, the laser treatment is used through a contact
lens which is mirrored to the angle of the eye. Microscopic
laser beams are then burnt to the angle, allowing the
aqueous fluid to exit the drainage canals better. Laser
trabeculoplasty is mostly accomplished in two sessions set
apart by a couple of weeks or months depending on the
swiftness of healing.

As a result of the treatment, the improved pathway of
drainage will potentially last only a couple of years, in which
time the drainage canals will have the tendency to clog up
again.

There are two various types of laser trabeculoplasty. One
of which is selective laser trabeculoplasty or SLT, and argon
laser trabeculoplasty or ALT. SLT is the least likely to leave
any scarring therefore this procedure can be repeated a
number of times, whereas ALT is not usually done again
after the second procedure (or session) because of how the

angle prevents scar tissue from healing as well. SLT on the other had is a procedure that can be repeated because of the significant absence of producing scarring in the angle.

But observation has determined that additional treatments after previous attempts have failed showed that success is low. So the options left to a patient would be to increase their usage of eye drops or get surgery. Ciliary body destruction or cyclophotocoagulation, more commonly known as laser cyclo-ablation is a procedure typically meant for patients who display severe forms of glaucoma and below than favorable visual potential.

Involving this procedure is the application of laser burns to the area of the eye which develops the aqueous fluid of the ciliary body. What this treatment therapy does is it destroys the cells which produce the fluid which in turn reduces the pressure to the eye. This form of laser procedure is usually done to a patient only when other sort of more traditional therapies have failed. Another method to achieve the same results of reducing aqueous fluid production is Cyclocryopexy. Cyclocryopexy is a method of freezing, in place of laser to come to a more limited amount of aqueous fluid.

Chapter Four: Unconventional Treatments for Glaucoma

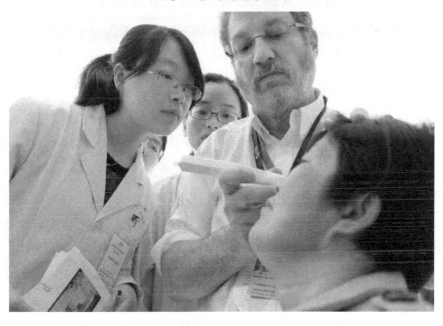

Glaucoma is an eye disease that interrupts the function of the optic nerve and if not arrested could be the cause for complete loss of vision in a person. Although the disease typically comes with age and is not accompanied by symptomatic pain, anyone regardless of age can succumb to the blinding truth about glaucoma when it is too late. With glaucoma being the second leading cause of population blindness in the world, and with the frequent side effects of many commercially available drugs, people have been looking more into the supplementary, alternative, and herbal remedies to help preserve and maintain an equilibrium of wellness. Our ability to expand research on medical topics has expanded and contracted in ways that are astounding to the times we live in. And yet, there are certain time tested methods, as well as food, that helps sustain and improve our health which is undeniable.

Aside from leading a healthy lifestyle, which we shall be discussing further later in the next chapter, what you put in your body - as in, what you eat - can go either way for your overall health. That much we all know. Take for example the man who, as fit as a fiddle, went on a mind bending, body re-shaping quest, eating only cheeseburgers and soda for a month, just to prove how awful we treat ourselves in terms of what we eat or the one who purposely put on the pounds documenting his journey, with the intent to see how hard it would be for an overweight person to get rid of poundage. Point being, whatever we take in, reflects, affects, and changes our chemistry and function.

Each one of us are made up differently on the microscopic, genetic and biological level, hence, you will have to work with your doctor to find the best herbal remedies to use with what has been prescribed to you. At any rate, many if not all the listed remedies and herbs here have proven their efficacy in maintain the health of humans and continue to bring great benefits to wellness.

Knowing what foods are healthy is important for us to know and observe as this is one way we can take control over our health and betterment. Knowing what to avoid, not only in the lifestyle we lead, that could deter our health and safety are things we need to know on the imperative in order to take back the rein of steering our health back to its optimum best.

More and more people have been looking into alternative treatments and have researched the ways and methods that were thought and proven to better health using natural sources from nature. The big pharma companies have cornered a market on research and development of supplementary, generic, therapeutic, and topical medicines using ancient herbal remedies as components in their manufactured drugs.

Find out more about the natural, holistic and alternative solutions nature has had for us for millennia and beyond, and discover a better way of gaining back your wellness. As with anything and everything related to your health, we are all individuals who react differently to what we ingest.

What is good for the goose is not always good for the gander. Be sure to consult with your doctor before trying out any of the recommended alternatives below since some medications given by your physician can react adversely when mixed with specific herbal remedies and vice versa. And since no two people are made up alike, what can work for one can be disastrous for another. Talk to your GP, and a last piece of advice, everything in moderation is the key.

Power Foods and Herbs - Stave Off Glaucoma Effects

Spinach, carotenoid and vitamin A are essential nutrients to help arrest glaucoma. Both of these sources of nutrients help improve the health of the retina and eye tissues. It is also recommended for glaucoma patients to take other green, leafy veggies. Lutein and xeaxanthin contained in these greens show to serve beneficial sustenance and nourishment to the eyes. Some excellent sources of these are kale, broccoli, collard greens, and brussel sprouts.

Egg yolks, raw ones in particular contain equal amounts of lutein and another cartenoid, zeaxanthin. These two together have shown great promise in the protection and preservation of eye sight.

Eating some healthy fats with your veggies allows the lutein to be absorbed better by your system, thereby maximizing its healing properties. So be sure to have your leafy greens with a little oil or butter for better internal reception.

Poach your eggs or cook them sunny side up and a little runny, because once the egg is cooked most of the essential nutrients you need is obliterated by heat and thorough cooking. Try consuming an organic egg by whipping it up to a shake as an alternative to semi-cooked eggs for better effects.

Avoid trans - fats at all costs as these interfere with the omega-3 fats you ingest. A high trans – fat diet has been suspected to contribute to macular damage. Trans - fat is contained and used in many foods like baked goods which have shortening and margarine. It is found in crackers, doughnuts, pastries, fried chicken and French fries. Allow the magic of Omega-3 fatty acid to do its work best by avoiding trans – fat.

Bioflavonoids from dark colored berries such as cranberries and blueberries are beneficial because of their properties that strengthen the capillaries responsible for transmitting nutrients to our eyes and throughout our body. Bilberry has been lauded for its properties that help prevent and reverse the damaging effects of macular degeneration. Eat berries in moderation as they do contain natural sugar. Having too much may interfere with your insulin levels.

One of the easiest available home remedies to arrest glaucoma is Fennel; adding a good measure of fennel to your daily serving of green salad to rid yourself of the pressure created in the eye caused by glaucoma. Alternately, you can chew fennel seeds as well. Fennel herb can also be boiled in water like you would tea. You can drink it like tea or you can cool down the tea and use it as eyewash twice a day for best results. Either way it is a great, readily available herb that can alleviate the pressure in the eye.

Eyebright Herb extracts is a natural herb that works great wonders against glaucoma. The extract of the herb can be applied directly to the eye with the use of a clean dropper. The efficacy of eyebright herb is astoundingly impressive and is one of the main components medicine manufacturers use to create eye drops.

Nutrients from the bilberry fruit helps to give protection to the retina from outside environmental factors of every day we can't avoid like the rays of the sun and dust. It ensures the optic nerve is properly functioning despite the harmful environment most of live in. After the consumption of bilberries, the pressure of the eye is soon released, easing the work and function of the optic nerve. In addition, the fruit is also been said to aid in the prevention of cataracts in old age.

Jaborandi is a rare, potent herb which grows and is found only in rainforest. It is natural herb whose extracts is said to be able to help restore vision wellness if used during the early stages of the retina displaying opacity. Jaborandi contains the nutrient pilocarpine and has been used in the manufacture of commercial eye products for over a century in human history.

Gingko biloba is a herb which releases oxygen in a person's system upon consumption. What ginko biloba specifically does is it flushes out the toxins which are harmfully settled in the eye tissues, arresting the any further damage of glaucoma and arresting any onset of it. The use of zinc sulfate along with gingko biloba has been lauded by some to avoid permanent blindness.

Collagen and Glaucoma

Fish Oil Omega-3 fatty acid found in wild caught fish has great benefits to the overall wellness and visual competency of the eyes. Not only does it protect eye health it also improves it. Tuna and salmon are great sources of fish oil omega-3 fatty acids. Prepare, serve up and have either of the fish four times a week and start up on the road to vision wellness and glaucoma arrest. You may also choose to substitute commercially available fish oil to do the job. Omega-3 fatty acid found in salmon, tuna, wild fish, and commercially prepared fish oils help in keeping the retina clear as well as restore normalcy in vision in people who are visually impaired.

Vitamin C is a proven medicine that is essential for everyone. Save for those who are allergic to citrus, people who have history of glaucoma in the family or those already suffering from it should have their daily intake of vitamin C. People in general are recommended a daily intake of at least 250mg of vitamin C for EVERY POUND of their body weight. Intake of the proper amount of vitamin c daily gives great benefit to the patient bearing glaucoma. It releases the pressure made by and to the optic nerve caused by glaucoma. Vitamin C has also been noted to promote good and better vision for those who have their regular proper serving.

Chapter Five: Managing Glaucoma with Better Lifestyle

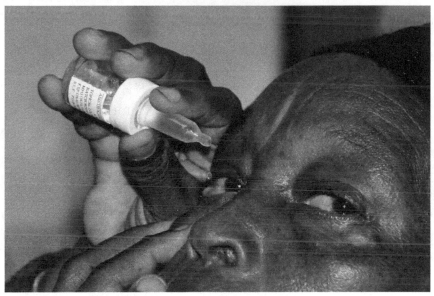

Aside from getting regular eye examinations, (please refer to our recommended list of scheduled eye exams above) eating the proper sorts of foods, getting the correct nutrients, and regular monitoring of your vision wellness, there are additional things we can do in order to improve our health. Not enough documentation is available on the impacts of lifestyle to a glaucoma patient, but sense and sensibilities not only tell us, but prove, that lifestyle can be a cause of the effect of glaucoma.

Hence, changing it up would be a wise idea, not only for those who suffer from it (who would most benefit), but also for those with history of glaucoma in the family. Simple mundane everyday things we do and take for granted, whether we like it or not, have medical impacts to us.

Lifestyle choices has its effects on IOP and largely owing to the fact that glaucoma is the second most frequent cause of blindness in the world, these have been documented well in several studies. Knowing how you can help yourself to avoid or manage glaucoma will be beneficial not only for you but also for friends or family members who may have or have possibility to develop glaucoma.

Some studies have been specifically focused on IOP. These studies have shown a stark correlation between vigorous exercise and the lowering of IOP in young adults. Smoking has some effects on chronic IOP elevation but there is no evidence to show that smoking is a risk for POAG. The correlation between IOP and diet is not just as clear as we would fancy it to be, but work is constantly underway to get to know more about glaucoma.

Glaucoma is becomes very severe especially if there is high and uncontrolled eye pressure. A reduction of the blood flow to the optic nerve at the back of the patient's eyes is another reason for its worsening. Therefore, it makes sense that there are things we do that causes an increase or decrease in eye pressure. Hypertension might also have an effect too.

Having huge amounts of caffeine raises ones IOP. Of course, that is not good news for patients who love coffee. If you intake about 5 or more cups a day or if the illness runs in the family, coffee drinkers as well as people who take in caffeinated drinks, increase their risk of glaucoma.

Many physicians just advise there glaucoma patients to drink coffee in utter moderation. It is also recommended that you avoid any sort of caffeine before you go in for a doctor's appointment because drinking anything with caffeine can surely affect your IOP score.

Are you a yoga enthusiast? Not all of us are but if you are well, this one is for you. Keep in mind that any position that has your heart above your head causes the IOP in your eye to elevate. So, if you have glaucoma and you stand on your head, STOP. Any position has your heart located higher than your head, you will have to forego.

As it turns out, even having pure water can elevate your IOP, it can usually affect your condition if you drink huge amounts of water in just a matter of minutes. All we need is a sufficient amount of water to stay healthy, so don't be put off by it. You will just need to spread your water intake throughout the day.

Apparently everyday mundane things like, playing a wind instrument, lifting weights, wearing a tight necktie or a pair of snug goggles all gives possibility to elevate IOP temporarily. But no proof of these activities making glaucoma worse has been noted. If you do have an advanced case of glaucoma, you may want to make some lifestyle changes just to be on the safe side.

What are things that could lower IOP then? Exercise is a double edged sword but if you know what to do, you can likely help yourself by doing what is right. Intense exercise can certainly do well to reduce IOP. On the other hand, it is also likely to lower blood pressure hence the supply to the optic nerve. So be mindful of your blood pressure when you are exercising.

Keep your blood pressure in check always as either high or low blood pressure are linked to damage of the optic nerve, most especially so if your blood pressure has the tendency to go down often overnight. Your position and how you lay in bed could also be linked to lowering or increasing your IOP. Resting or sleeping with your head propped on a pillow lessens the IOP. However do not bury your eye on your pillow to maintain correct flow.

A modest and very moderate amount of alcohol could have some benefits in lowering IOP. On the other hand, excessive intake of alcohol, along with other adverse effect, damages the optic nerve. So be frugal about how you accept alcoholic beverages.

There are no specific recommendations to take or not to take dietary supplements. Although Omega-3 oils are largely beneficial for eye health in general, not a single person has yet identified what will either aid or be detrimental for glaucoma patients.

Gingko bilboa does merit special mention though because of the herbal extract properties that it has which is thought to improve the flow of blood to the optic nerve as it does throughout the body. It has been seen to be a potential agent for neuron protection and short-term visual field improvement when used by patients who suffer from normal-tension glaucoma.

It is a powerful and organic product which can be mixed with other medicines you may be taking and it is highly likely that it will not go well for everyone. Make it a point to talk to your GP or your ophthalmologist before taking gingko bilboa. Also, ginko bilboa lessens of the ability of blood to clot well so anyone taking gingko bilboa should stop before they go into surgery of any sort.

A diet rich in magnesium, omega-3 and omega-6 fatty acids and dark chocolate correlates to better blood flow overall. Antioxidants such as melatonin and flavonoids found in tea, red wine and coffee may lessen the mitochondrial oxidative stress. Again, a word of caution, everything should be in moderation. Keep in mind that too much caffeine will elevate IOP drastically.

Alternative Medicine

Before trying any form of alternative remedies, make sure to consult with your doctor. Some herbal medicine recommended by alternative medicine can be highly toxic, difficult to find in its raw form and may be illegal to transport without permit. Others forms of Ayuverdic or Chinese medicine in pill or capsule form have only been approved as supplements with no healing guarantees.

Chinese or Oriental medicine looks to combinations of herbal remedies that make up topical ointments, tonics, elixirs, eye drops that are largely unavailable in Western countries but reportedly work better than most pharmacy medications for glaucoma. Acupuncture is also used to relieve pressure of fluid in the eye.

Ayuverdic the ancient Indian system of medicine has used the combination of health beneficial, potent herbs found in nature which help strengthen our bodies, build endurance, and improve one's immunity. This natural system of using herbs to maintain wellness has been reported to do wonders for those with glaucoma by using the most effective herbs.

Keep in mind that you want to take caution about not heeding your doctor's orders on taking your prescribed medicine. Self-medicating should be avoided at all costs since glaucoma is a lifelong disease that will need proper monitoring, maintenance and medication. Vision impairment and blindness is not a joke and should be given the proper attention and treatment if you want to enjoy the gift of sight for a long time to come.

Living with Glaucoma

A glaucoma patient will generally be asked to make some lifestyle changes like limiting or eliminating cigarette smoking. They would be told that exercising on a regular basis will help lower IOP. They will be advised strongly to put a cap on their caffeine intake, and they would be told to avoid positions where they have their head down (remember? heart higher than head positions?).

We have compiled a list of foods you may want to avoid or at the very least cut down intake as this can greatly reduce your chances of worsening your glaucoma condition. As with everything that has been mentioned, take everything in moderation but do pay mind to things that you know will either increase your blood pressure or things that may affect your IOP.

Avoid any foods that you know cause you allergic reactions. Food allergies could be highly responsible for placing pressure on the eyes, so pay mind about what foods have this effect on you.

Caffeine is one that is high on this list of foods to avoid for glaucoma patients and those who have family members who have the destructive eye disease. Not only would those who do not have glaucoma but have susceptibility for it be able to make better choices about their continued health, patients experiencing glaucoma would be able to help arrest the deterioration. And along with treatment and regular monitoring they could well save their eyesight.

Apart from the one glass of red wine, which can actually help with the increase of blood flow in some glaucoma cases, alcohol consumption most especially in great amounts can lead to liver toxicity. So those already suffering from glaucoma would be better off taking heed about how much alcohol they should limit themselves.

Chapter Six: Preserving the Gift of Sight

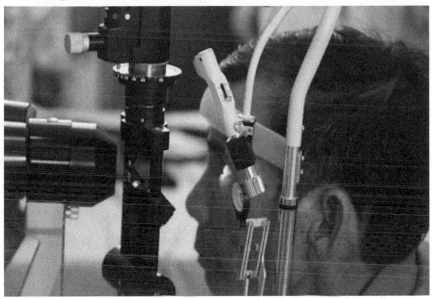

Do you exercise to stay healthy and in shape? Do you study in order to learn? Do you protect your property home and family? If you answered yes to anyone of them, then be thankful that you could read that. We all make it a point to protect our property, acquisitions and finances, but for what purpose, if we cannot enjoy it due to ill - wealth? This is to say that we do things to improve ourselves, protect ourselves, and the material things we collect but why do so many of neglect to protect our eye sight? Many people take their wellness for granted and leave it to fate to get them by.

Much like breathing we take our ability to see as a matter of fact. But think about it, the eye is one part of our body the most exposed to the elements which is located both in and out of our body.

It is comprised of thin membranes, glutinous gel like substances, clear lenses, the optic nerve, canals and channels, vessels and material which make up this amazing organ that allows us the gift of sight. We do not come with spare parts. Our eyes are irreplaceable and they deserve the attention and care because of the many benefits it adds to our quality of life. The advances in medical science and technology have given human beings the ability to study and learn things that have advanced modern medicine and have propelled it to greater heights than ever before.

Along with the other parts of our bodies, the eyes are a pretty well-worked piece of machinery that allows us to see. There are many factors that put our eyes and our eye sight at risk of injury or inherited eye conditions, as glaucoma sometimes may be for some.

Environmental conditions, like exposure to the sun, dust, wind, heavy metal rain, as well as being in the constant presence of your computer, laptop, mobile or TV screen are just some of the added negative impact that wreak havoc on the condition and wellness of our eyes and eyesight.

Individuals would usually go to see their doctor about their visual condition only when damage is apparent, when there is a sudden injury or when visual impairment is experienced. Sometimes it could be too late to do anything about it.

The Importance of Routine Eye Checkup

African Americans and Asians have a greater likelihood of developing glaucoma than Caucasians. The premise is that people of a particular heritage and diversities with smaller eyes run a higher risk of contracting, developing and having glaucoma than their Caucasian counterparts.

Open-angle glaucoma is the most common form of glaucoma when the drainage canals of the eyes get choked up through time. This is what causes the intraocular pressure to increase because the proper amount of fluid is not being drained from the eye.

With the advances of what we know about the body, specifically the eyes, and the great propulsion medical technology has driven us to knowing more about sight preservation, methods, techniques. Tools have been created and improved throughout time to allow doctors to see into the eye in order to make diagnosis. Peering into our dilated eyes, doctors can now tell the wellness of our eyes. They can detect the slightest abnormalities and changes within the core of our eyes.

Computerized scanners are now able to spot blood vessels that are ready to inundate the retina. A device is now used in order to find starving sight cells by the mere analysis of the density of the retina's color. There is another device that is able to identify potential blind spots before it happens. Some of these devices are high tech and advanced whilst others are simple low-tech equipment used and improved through our advance in science.

Aside from the medical machines and gadgetry which allow doctors to peer into the windows of our being, pharmaceuticals have been able to come up with medicine in aid of treatment, there are now anesthetic eye drops that help ensure a fairly comfortable and painless experience during examinations.

The advantage of getting a routine checkup is that you are administered exams worthy of the service your eyes give you. These tests are not only able to document the conditions and the mechanisms of your eyes, these regular eye examinations can detect chronic eye diseases and arrest them. Even though no cures yet exist, these tests, at the very least can possibly arrest the further damage eye diseases, like glaucoma can create. It potentially delays any more significant sight loss.

With treatments, medicine and technology being developed exponentially and the rate of new drugs saving the eye sight of millions of people, there is no reason not to take better care of your sight. With the recent success in gene therapy, we are getting closer and closer to cures more than prevention. In addition there are hundreds of clinical trials being carried out all over the globe in the development drugs and treatment to intervene with glaucoma onset.

Chapter Seven: Treatment and Wellness

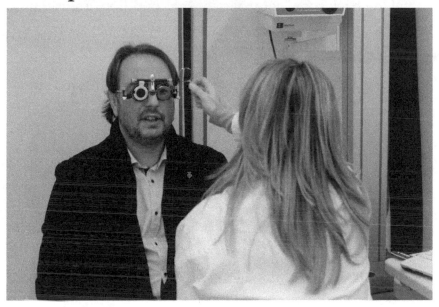

The knowledge of having a chronic health condition like glaucoma which can potentially rob you of your ability to see has its psychological and emotional impacts that are overwhelming to a person. Upon understanding the implications of the degenerative eye condition, a person who is diagnosed with glaucoma may begin to go through anxiety, fear, feeling helpless, lethargy or depression. These are valid feeling that typically hounds anyone who is given news of this magnitude.

Knowing more about the disease is one good way of taking back some control over the condition. Taking time to understand what the condition is, what the implications are, the available medication and treatments are just some ways for a glaucoma patient to take back some control over the condition.

Join support groups and network for support. Again, therapy and medication that works for one does not necessarily mean it will work for all. Networking with support groups allow you and family members to understand more of the disease, get updated about breakthroughs in medicine and treatment methods and even cure.

Learning more about the disease will allow you to discover steps on how to manage and control the situation because you would be able to know what you can do to arrest any further damage.

Even patients with low vision have been able to work with rehab counselors for them to be able to lead fairly active lives. There are some workarounds you can discuss with your rehab counselor that can help in lead a good quality of life even after diagnosis.

Diagnosing glaucoma is not typically easy to make, therefore careful study and monitor of the optic nerve continues to be an essential part to the diagnosis and treatment a patient gets. Make sure to schedule regular eye examination with your doctors to rule out glaucoma each time.

The most important factor of concern is the protection of a patient's sight. Doctors look at a number of factors before they make any conclusions or decisions about the patient's treatment.

The buildup of aqueous fluid pressure occurs slowly in the most common type of glaucoma and often not accompanied by any pain or outwardly symptom to give suspect. The less common glaucoma forms are in fact accompanied by more telling symptoms such as headaches, eye aches, and the appearance of rainbows around bright lights, vomiting, nausea, hazy vision or sudden sight loss. There are secondary forms of glaucoma that require immediate medical attention.

There is no cure yet for glaucoma but studies, research and advancements in medicine are geared toward improving the knowledge of the causes and prevention of glaucoma. Improving treatments are also well underway as studies get closer to revealing more about what cures can be administered.

Most medications are accompanied by side effect and will usually pester out after a couple of weeks. It is important that you are told about any emotional or physical changes you may experience upon taking medication geared toward treatment of glaucoma. You have to proactively offer information about any effects of the medication given to your physician. Older people are especially reminded to be aware of any changes in their mobility or behavior which could be side effects of the medication you have been given because if this becomes a problem for the patient the doctor may just change the treatment option or medication.

A change of medication has to be expected and does not immediately equate that the glaucoma is getting the best of you. It is normal for doctors to change up the glaucoma medication due to the ultimate development for tolerance of your body to the drug. When this happens, the medication will lose efficacy. Doctors will typically go full circle sometimes and prescribe medicines previously given to you.

Follow the medication regimen to a tee to be able to see improvements. Be compliant about it and develop the discipline of taking them when you should. Surgery can only do so much, as you have learnt here, and medication can only work if administered properly at the proper times. Face it, much of the responsibility of your eye care falls on your shoulders and medications can only work properly so long as they are used in the prescribed manner.

Stay on track and make a schedule on a planner that is visible like on your office desk, on the refrigerator door, or log it on your phone where it can alert you for when you should take administer. Be sure to include the dosage and name of the medication to be administered. You can use little colored stickers to help you identify them just make sure they are labeled according to their color.

Should you miss out on one eye drop administration, apply them as soon as you remember. Make sure that you are doing it correctly by first allowing your doctor to show you which part of the eye you should be applying. Do one better and show your doctor how you administer the eye drop so they can give you directives if needed.

When taking more than three of any sort of medication, regardless of target, including vitamins, supplements and natural remedies, discuss this with your pharmacist or doctor as one or the other may interact negatively to each other.

The easiest way to put in eye drops in the eye is for you to sit with your head tilted back. You can also lie on your back and put in the drops. Make sure that you wash your hands before administering eye drops;

- Pull the lower lid of your eye creating a cup.
- Look up and squeeze one drop into the cupped low lid of your eye. Do not attempt to wipe away the medication, touch your eye or blink.
- Avoid the tip of the spout from touching your eye, nor should the spout tip touch any part of your face, skin or eyes.
- Once the medicine is in, close your eyes for about 2-3 minutes and let it start to absorb for it to do its job.
- Do this for both eyes, waiting 3-5 minutes in between the next drop if more than one is necessary. This ensures that whichever was administered first will do its job as with the second medication after.
- Should you have trouble getting the eye drop in your eye, try lying down flat on your back. With your face

up and your eyes closed place one drop outside the corners of your eyes near the bridge of your nose. When you have placed drops on each, open your eyes and the drops should fall in.

- Make sure that enough of the solution has been placed in your eyes and did not just roll off your skin.

Should you notice changes in your vision like loss of contrast sensitivity, light sensitivity, reduced vision, or problems with glare, let your doctor know. Some patients suffering from glaucoma experience low vision even with the aid of contact lenses or glasses, making every day routines more challenging.

Some of these activities may include driving, getting around, and other daily regimens. There are a number of workarounds like using magnifying glasses, colored lenses when the ability to see shades of similar colors is impaired as well as text enlargers which come with some computers.

Make sure that you have at least two bottles of the same medicine available in places where you are usually, like in the office and at home. This ensures that you will be able to take your medication no matter where you are.

Let your healthcare providers know if you have been given medication to treat another condition. You don't want one reacting negatively with another. Make sure that the medications you take for other conditions are not interfering with glaucoma medications. Be wary of any medication containing steroid.

Make sure that you always get an exam before going on long trips or starting anything long term. Make sure that your doctor knows of any changes in your schedule as they may help in rescheduling your intake of medication.

Write down any questions you may have about your condition and be sure to discuss them the next time you meet with your doctor. And before you leave your doctor's office make your next appointment and make sure you write this down.

Keep your eyes clean and protect them from irritants. Wear protective goggles when swimming or when doing yard work, most especially after eye surgery. Do not attempt to rub or scratch them even when tickled or itchy.

Women are especially reminded to be mindful of the type of cosmetics they use and use non-hypoallergenic products. Replacing your eye cosmetics frequently without prolonged usage is another way to save your eyes from unwanted irritation.

Eat healthy foods, and take care of the rest of your body. Maintaining overall good health is as important as taking care of your peepers. Stay at a healthy weight, exercise regularly, quit smoking, cut down on the caffeine intake and sleep well. Remember that eye strain can be uncomfortable. Staring at your computer screen or TV for long stretches of time creates great strain not only to your eyes but to your eye sight as well. Give your eyes a break by resting them periodically.

Should the condition of the patient be particularly difficult to diagnose or treat, they may be referred to a glaucoma specialist. Getting a second opinion is always wise. This is especially expressed if the patient or doctor become concerned about the given diagnosis or progress.

Bonus Chapter:
Famous People Who Have Glaucoma

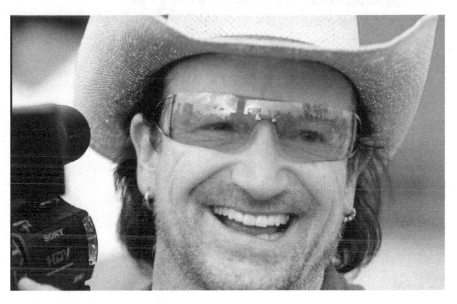

The American Academy of Ophthalmologists states that half the population of Americans suffering from glaucoma does not know about this silent condition or are even aware that they have it. No one is spared from glaucoma. Young or old, man or woman, everyday people and celebrities alike are all at risk to develop one sort of glaucoma or another. The only way to arrest the damages brought on by glaucoma is to get your eyes examined regularly.

An individual who has glaucoma in the family history as well as some select people of certain ethnicity are encouraged to have more frequent exams.

We have compiled a short list of famous celebrities who have been suffering from one form of glaucoma or another to show the indiscriminate "selection" of the damaging and irreversible effects of glaucoma.

#1: Ray Charles Robinson

American singer-songwriter, musician, and composer

Known For: Known as "The Genius," hit songs include "Hit the Road, Jack," "Georgia on My Mind," "Seven Spanish Angels"

Charles began noticing anomalies with his vision and began to lose sight when he was 5 years old. Although never confirmed by the impressive singer/musician, untreated glaucoma is suspected to be the reason why he became completely blind by the time he reached the age of seven. Given the era he was born into, when many things were unknown in medicine, not to mention their economic background, there was little him or his mother could do to stop the progression of the vision-robbing disease. Poverty gave them no access to treatment which could have.

These days childhood glaucoma is often treated, corrected and managed through a procedure called filtering microsurgery. This operation creates a new drainage passage for the fluid to exit.

#2: Andrea Bocelli

Italian Singer – Songwriter, Classical and Opera singer, Recording Artist

Known For: "Because We Believe," "The Prayer," "Vivo Per Lei," "Time to Say Goodbye," "Somos Novios"

The multi-million record selling tenor, Andrea Bocelli gave special mention to his mother, Edi, in the middle of his concert in Italy and thanked her for going against doctors wishes of aborting him when he was in utero. Bocelli's mother, whilst pregnant with him had to undergo appendectomy and was later advised by doctors to get an abortion. His mother resisted the advice and had him a few months later. Andrea was diagnosed with congenital glaucoma when he was born. With his eyesight already being at a risk because of his condition, the tenor from Italy went totally blind at 12 years old when he suffered a brain hemorrhage after a football accident.

Congenital glaucoma is a rare form of glaucoma which can be hereditary. Some children grow up only to, later on, develop the condition. Indications of childhood glaucoma would be sensitivity to light, profuse tearing and a cloudy cornea.

#3: Bono

Irish Rock Star, Singer – songwriter, Lead Vocalist of Rock Band called U2. He's also a venture capitalist and philantrophist.

Known For: "With or Without You," "You're the Best Thing About Me," "One" "Beautiful Day," Sweetest Thing"

U2 front man, Bono, once revealed in a 2014 interview that he has been living with glaucoma for over 20 years. This was his response to Graham Norton's query about why he was never seen without glasses. Bono thought it was an opportune time to talk about his condition adding that he has been getting properly treated and that he was going to be fine.

The eyes of people who suffer from glaucoma are very sensitive to glaring lights and given recommendation to wear sunshades. The Glaucoma Research Foundation recommends a pair of sunshades that blocks 99 to 100 percent of UV rays.

#4: Former U.S. Senator John Glenn

U.S. Marine Corps Aviator, Engineer, Astronaut, U.S. Senator from Ohio

Known For: John Glenn is the first man to orbit the earth, and he also served as a U.S. Senator from 1987 – 1995.

One of the most convincing cases for advocating early glaucoma detection is US Senator John Glenn. If not for early detection the first man who orbited the Earth would not have enjoyed further exploration of space if not for early detection and proper treatment. Astronaut Glenn urged Americans and raised glaucoma awareness in a 2002 public service campaign where he urged Americans to understand and get tested for glaucoma.

Dilated, comprehensive eye exams, once every two to four years are strongly recommended for adults over 40. People over 60 should get their eyes tested and monitored at least once a year.

#5: Whoopi Goldberg

American comedian, singer, and actress, T.V. Host, author

Known For: "Sister Act movies," "Ghost," "Lion King" Host of "The View." Best – selling author of If Someone Says, "You Complete Me," RUN!

Comedian and actress, Whoopi Goldberg, revealed in 2014 that she used marijuana by way of vaporizers to help alleviate glaucoma symptoms. Marijuana is commonly known to help ease symptoms of glaucoma. Goldberg, suffering from painful headaches said that marijuana reduced the discomfort of the condition.

The Glaucoma Research Foundation states that no studies have been done to prove the efficacy of medical marijuana use in reducing eye pressure any better than commercially available medications. Glaucoma comes with symptoms like, nausea, vomiting, blurred vision, eye pain and headaches.

#6: Kirby Puckett

American Major League Baseball Player, Baseball Hall of Famer, Center Fielder for Minnesota Twins

Known For: World Series Champion, ALCS MVP

Kirby Puckett was a Hall of Fame baseball player with the Minnesota Twins and who helped the team win two World Series titles in the late 80s and early 90s. One morning in 1996, the then 36 year old center fielder, which held all-time leader in career hits, runs and bases, woke up blind in one eye. He was diagnosed with central retinal vein occlusion, a form of glaucoma, which sped up his retirement. Glaucoma symptoms are silent and unassuming. Most people do not know they have the disease until it has progressed. For this reason, it is highly imperative to get regular dilated eye exams. If caught during the early stages, eye drops or pills can help manage glaucoma.

Index

L

M

N

O

P

R

Photo References

Page 8 Photo by user TobiasD via Pixabay.com,
https://pixabay.com/en/eye-human-face-vision-look-person-321961/

Page 12 Photo by user Community Eye Health via Flicker.com,
https://www.flickr.com/photos/communityeyehealth/8438911894/

Page 25 Photo by user TEDx SanDiego via Flicker.com,
https://www.flickr.com/photos/tedxsandiego/8253376939/

Page 36 Photo by user Community Eye Health via Flicker.com,
https://www.flickr.com/photos/communityeyehealth/8437824353/

Page 61 Photo by user Orbis via Flicker.com,
https://www.flickr.com/photos/orbis_emea/13886992412/

Page 70 Photo by user Community Eye Health via Flicker.com,
https://www.flickr.com/photos/communityeyehealth/8437828857/

Page 79 Photo by user Orbis via Flicker.com,
https://www.flickr.com/photos/orbis_emea/5706979305/

Page 85 Photo by user Premsa SantCugat via Flicker.com,
https://www.flickr.com/photos/premsasantcugat/1218850318
3/

Page 95 Photo by user Danny Hammontree via Flicker.com,
https://www.flickr.com/photos/digitalgrace/63746104

References

Acute Angle-Closure Glaucoma - Emedicinehealth.com
https://www.emedicinehealth.com/acute_angle-closure_glaucoma/article_em.htm

Angle Recession Glaucoma – Medscape.com
https://emedicine.medscape.com/article/1204999-overview

Are You at Risk For Glaucoma? - Glaucoma.org
https://www.glaucoma.org/glaucoma/are-you-at-risk-for-glaucoma.php

Do Lifestyle Choices Affect Glaucoma? - Glaucoma.org
https://www.glaucoma.org/glaucoma/do-lifestyle-choices-affect-glaucoma.php

Eye Anatomy - Glaucoma.org
https://www.glaucoma.org/glaucoma/anatomy-of-the-eye.php

Home Remedies Glaucoma - HomeMadeMedicine.com
https://www.homemademedicine.com/home-remedies-glaucoma.html

Glaucoma facts - MedicineNet.com
https://www.medicinenet.com/glaucoma/article.htm#glaucoma_facts

Glaucoma Facts and Stats - Glaucoma.org
https://www.glaucoma.org/glaucoma/glaucoma-facts-and-stats.php

Lifestyle choices play important role in glaucoma management – Healio.com
https://www.healio.com/ophthalmology/glaucoma/news/print/ocular-surgery-news-europe-edition/%7B9e43aa67-d7ca-4e63-b4ad-75ae485fa9a7%7D/lifestyle-choices-play-important-role-in-glaucoma-management

Secondary Glaucomas - Glaucoma-Association.com
http://www.glaucoma-association.com/media/wysiwyg/Leaflet_PDF_Files/Secondary_Glaucoma.pdf

Symptoms of Open-Angle Glaucoma - Glaucoma.org
https://www.glaucoma.org/glaucoma/symptoms-of-primary-open-angle-glaucoma.php

Tonometry and Glaucoma - MedicineNet.com
https://www.medicinenet.com/tonometry/article.htm

Types of Glaucoma - Glaucoma.org
https://www.glaucoma.org/glaucoma/types-of-glaucoma.php

What are the Symptoms of Glaucoma? - Glaucoma.org
https://www.glaucoma.org/gleams/what-are-the-symptoms-of-glaucoma.php

What Is Glaucoma? – Healthline.com
https://www.healthline.com/health/glaucoma#overview1

What Is Glaucoma? – WebMD.com
https://www.webmd.com/eye-health/glaucoma-eyes#1

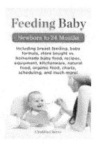

Feeding Baby
Cynthia Cherry
978-1941070000

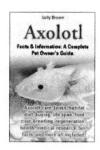

Axolotl
Lolly Brown
978-0989658430

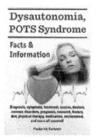

Dysautonomia, POTS
Syndrome
Frederick Earlstein
978-0989658485

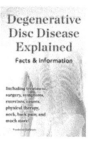

Degenerative Disc
Disease Explained
Frederick Earlstein
978-0989658485

Sinusitis, Hay Fever,
Allergic Rhinitis Explained
Frederick Earlstein
978-1941070024

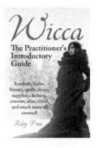

Wicca
Riley Star
978-1941070130

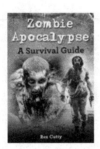

Zombie Apocalypse
Rex Cutty
978-1941070154

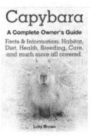

Capybara
Lolly Brown
978-1941070062

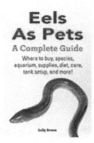

Eels As Pets
Lolly Brown
978-1941070167

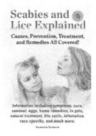

Scabies and Lice Explained
Frederick Earlstein
978-1941070017

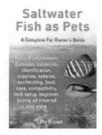

Saltwater Fish As Pets
Lolly Brown
978-0989658461

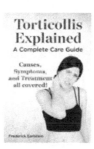

Torticollis Explained
Frederick Earlstein
978-1941070055

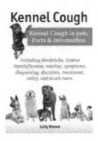

Kennel Cough
Lolly Brown
978-0989658409

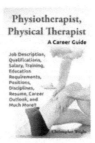

Physiotherapist, Physical
Therapist
Christopher Wright
978-0989658492

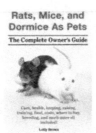

Rats, Mice, and Dormice
As Pets
Lolly Brown
978-1941070079

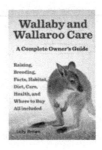

Wallaby and Wallaroo Care
Lolly Brown
978-1941070031

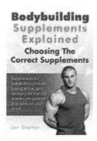

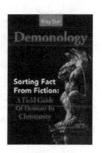

Bodybuilding Supplements
Explained
Jon Shelton
978-1941070239

Demonology
Riley Star
978-19401070314

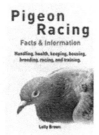

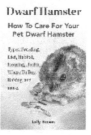

Pigeon Racing
Lolly Brown
978-1941070307

Dwarf Hamster
Lolly Brown
978-1941070390

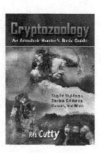

Cryptozoology
Rex Cutty
978-1941070406

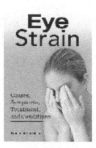

Eye Strain
Frederick Earlstein
978-1941070369

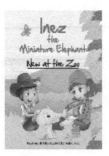

Inez The Miniature Elephant
Asher Ray
978-1941070353

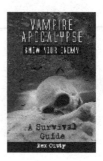

Vampire Apocalypse
Rex Cutty
978-1941070321